THE GANJA DICTIONARY

The layman's guide to nature's
most controversial herb

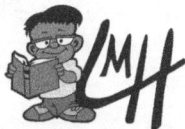

LMH PUBLISHING LIMITED

Compiled by: L. Mike Henry & K. Sean Harris
Cover concept by: K. Sean Harris
Cover Design by: Roshane Anglin
Typeset & Book Layout: Roshane Anglin

Published by: LMH Publishing Ltd.
Suite 10-11, Sagicor Industrial Park
7 Norman Road
Kingston C.S.O., Jamaica
Tel: 876-938-0005
Fax: 876-759-8752
Email: lmhbookpublishing@cwjamaica.com
Website: www.lmhpublishing.com

Printed in Canada   ISBN: 978-976-8245-68-7

NATIONAL LIBRARY OF JAMAICA CATALOGUING IN
PUBLICATION DATA
Henry, L. Mike
      The ganja dictionary: the layman's guide to nature's most
controversial
herb / L. Mike Henry.

     p. : ill. ; cm
ISBN 978-976-8245-68-7

1   Marijuana – Jamaica. 2. Marijuana – Therapeutic use.
3.   Marijuana – Physiological effects   4. Cannabis – Jamaica.
5. Ganja.
I.   Title

615.7827   dc 23

"The illegality of cannabis is outrageous, an impediment to full utilization of a drug which helps produce insight, sensitivity and fellowship so desperately needed in this increasingly mad and dangerous world."
Carl Sagan

DISCLAIMER

The author (s) and publisher do not directly or indirectly diagnose, dispense medical advice or prescribe the use of ganja as a form of treatment without medical approval. The intent is only to offer information. In the event you use this information without your doctor's approval, you are prescribing for yourself, which is your right, but the publisher and the author (s) assume no responsibility.

CONTENT

About Ganja

When many people hear the word ganja, they think of Rastafarianism, and erroneously think that the word is of Jamaican origin. It's actually a Sanksrit word and was commonly used in India to describe a specific, potent strain of sativa.

Also known as marijuana (Mexican name for the plant that became mainstream in the early 1900s), cannabis (the scientific term), weed (probably because of the plant's ability to sprout anywhere a seed finds itself) and many other terms across the world, ganja is arguably the world's most controversial herb. Legality is usually a matter of power, not justice or morality, and ganja's journey highlights that.

The US government passed the Marijuana Tax Act of 1937 that effectively banned the use and sale of ganja. Years later the Act was ruled unconstitutional and was replaced with the Controlled Substances Act in the 70s that established schedules for ranking substances according to their potential for addiction and how dangerous they were. Ganja was placed in the most restrictive schedule, schedule 1, which consists of drugs like LSD, ecstasy and heroin despite the proven value of the herb as a medicinal plant that could successfully be used in the treatment of cancer, glaucoma, arthritis, epilepsy, chronic pain, depression and a host of other medical issues.

The demonization of this remarkable herb has been a great disservice to the world. For over 5000 years ganja was viewed and used as a therapeutic agent worldwide, until the US government decided otherwise with the aforementioned Act in 1937. It is good to see that people are waking up worldwide, but of course, as with many things, it starts with the US. The state of California was the first state to approve the use of ganja for medical purposes (1996), and to date twenty-three states have passed medical marijuana laws, and the state of Colorado, where there are more dispensaries than coffee and fast food locations, allows its use for recreation. The ganja industry in the US is on track to post over 20 billion in sales by 2020.

As of 2017, countries like the Netherlands, Portugal, Spain, Uruguay, Canada and here in Jamaica, where it has been decriminalized and persons can carry up to two ounces and grow up to five plants per household, have the least restrictive ganja laws, while countries like Turkey, China, Egypt, France and the Philippines have the strictest ganja laws.

Brief History of Ganja

The earliest record of ganja was in the writings of the Chinese emperor Shen Nung dating 2737 BC. He mostly wrote about the herb's medicinal value, focusing on its use in the treatment of malaria, gout and rheumatism, and ironically, absent-mindedness (so much for its reputation as a cause of short-term memory loss).

Ganja was introduced to Jamaica in the 1850s-1860s by indentured servants. It became a mainstay on the island in short order, popular particularly among the poor working class. The Jamaican government enacted the Ganja Law of 1913, outlawing the herb despite its immense popularity. It did nothing to slow or stop the use of the herb. It only served to create an additional burden on the court system, and to allow for the incarceration of many people, especially those of the poor rural areas and the ghettoes of the major towns.

The Rastafarian movement concretized the ganja culture in Jamaica. For many Rastafarians, smoking ganja is a spiritual act, a sacrament that cleanses the body and mind, helps one to meditate, encourages peacefulness and brings them closer to the Most I (Jah). Rastafarians believe ganja to be sanctioned by the Bible as they consider it to be a part of the Tree of Life.

The movement to legalize ganja began in the 1960s, and at long last, almost sixty years later, there is progress as it has been decriminalized, as previously mentioned.

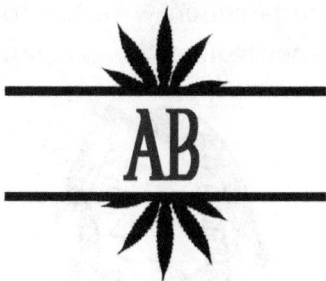

Baked: To be high from smoking ganja.

Big Head: A spliff rolled in such a manner that the end that will be lit (the head) is much larger than the rest of the spliff.

Blazed: Another term that refers to being high from smoking ganja.

Blunt: Ganja rolled with the tobacco-leaf wrapper from a cheap cigar. (illus.)

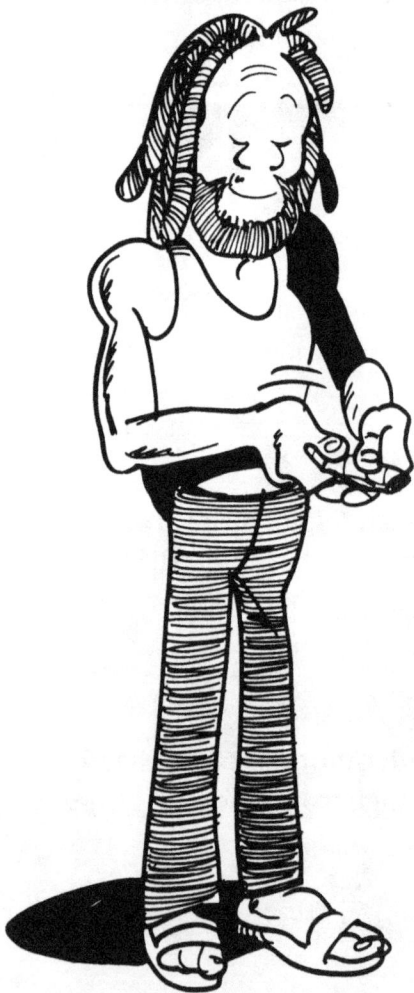

Bong: A water pipe used for smoking ganja. *(image)*

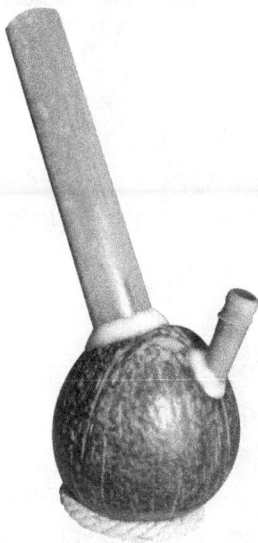

Bud: The flowers of the ganja plant. This is the part that is smoked.

Bush Weed: Ganja of inferior quality.

C

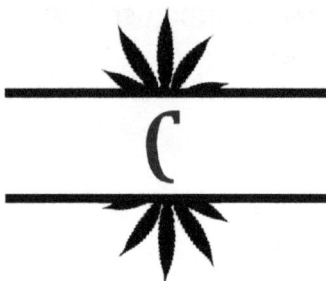

Chalice: A type of water pipe with a hose or draw-tube for inhaling. Often used by Rastafarians for spiritual practices.

Chillum Pipe: A type of hand pipe used for smoking ganja.

Crystals: Technically known as trichomes, they are the tiny sparkles on the ganja plant.

Cure: The process that gives the ganja its sweet smell and smoking qualities. It improves potency and makes the ganja less harsh.

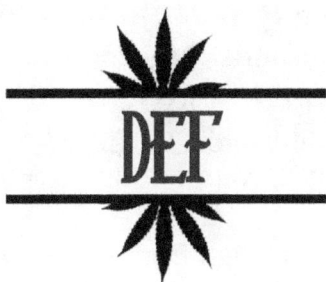

Edibles: Treats, savoury or sweet, that have been infused with ganja and are consumed orally to get high. Brownies are one of the most popular forms of edibles. *(image)*

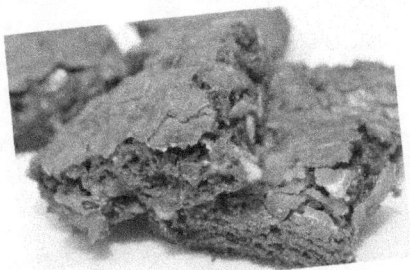

Fire: High quality ganja.

Four-twenty (4/20): April 20th, the day thousands of Americans (and others worldwide), celebrate the joys of ganja by officially indulging, often with friends in a group setting.

Frass: To be high from smoking ganja. (illus.)

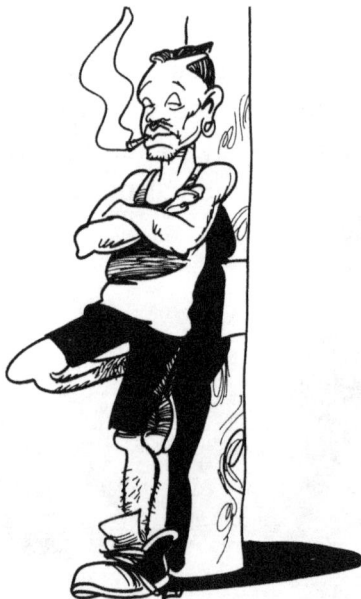

Fronto leaf: Wrapper grade tobacco leaf. The thicker, darker variety is popular in many Caribbean islands.

G

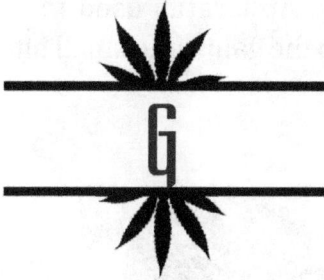

Ganja: A popular term (Sankrit origin) for the cannabis plant.

Grabba: Fronto leaf that is broken down into bits or strips and added to ganja for smoking. *(image)*

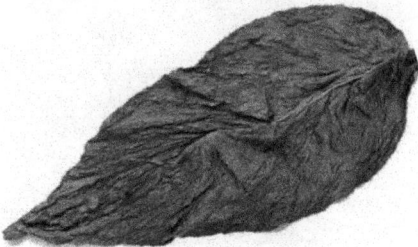

Grinder: Apparatus used to crush or break up the ganja into small bits. *(image)*

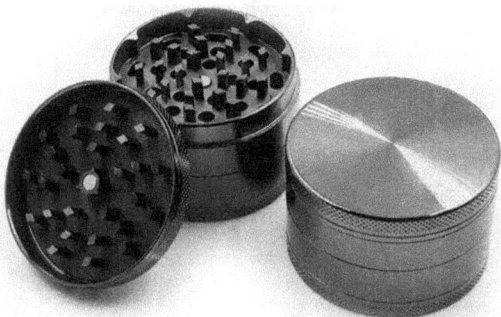

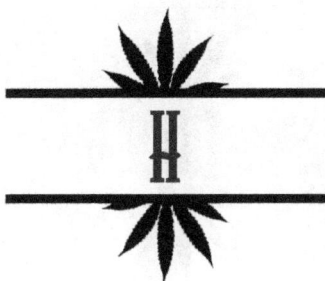

High: The effect from smoking or consuming ganja orally.

High Grade: Top quality ganja.

Hydro: Short for hydroponic, it is a plant-growing technique that does not require soil (water is used to deliver the plant's nutrients), and also refers to ganja grown by this method.

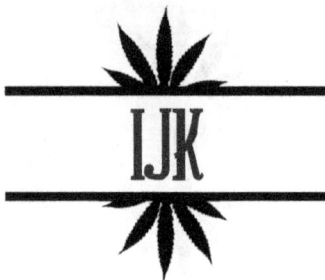

Indica: A strain of ganja known for its fat leaves and short flowering cycles. The effects of this strain tend to be more sedating than stimulating. *(image)*

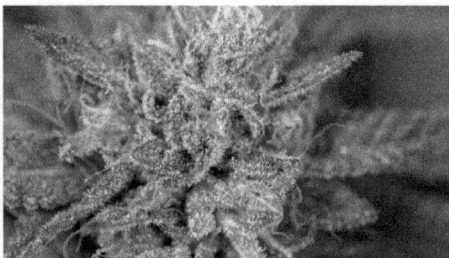

Indo: Ganja that is grown in perfect indoor conditions; high quality, pungent and powerful ganja. *(image)*

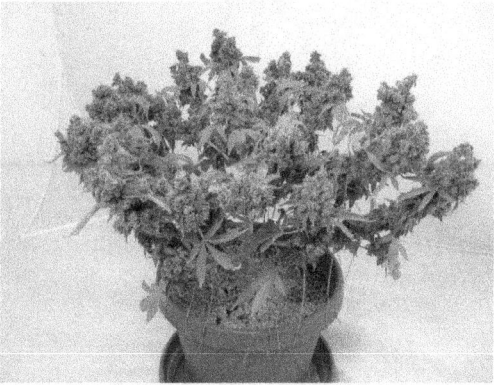

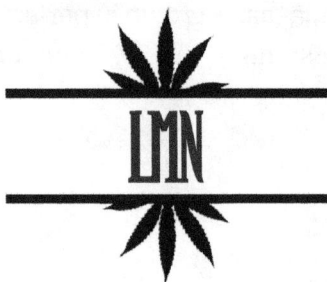

Marijuana: The cannabis plant, also known as ganja.

Mary Jane: Used to be an undercover way of referring to ganja but became so popular everyone now knows the reference.

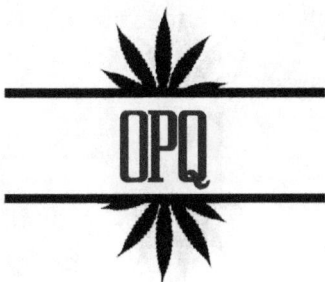

Pack a Bowl: To put ganja in a pipe for smoking.

Pot: Slang for ganja (mostly used by white Americans).

Pre-roll: A term mostly used by dispensaries to describe a spliff or joint.

RST

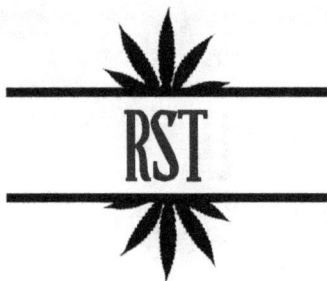

Reefer: Slang for ganja.

Rizzla: A brand of paper commonly used to roll spliffs.

Sensimilla: A seedless ganja plant.

Spliff: A ganja joint; also known as a marijuana cigarette. *(image)*

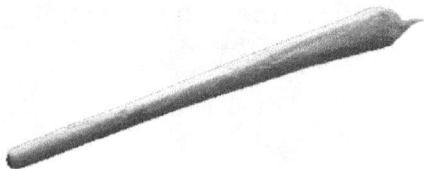

Spliff Tail: The tiny piece left when one smokes a spliff.

Sticky Icky: Really good ganja.

Stoner: An ardent indulger of smoking ganja.

Stoned: High from smoking ganja.

Toke: The act of physically inhaling ganja smoke.

Trees: Slang term for ganja. *(image)*

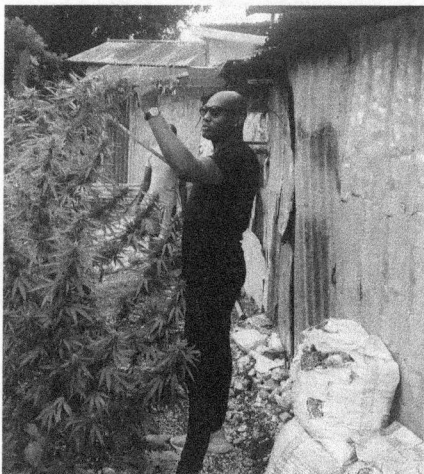

UVW

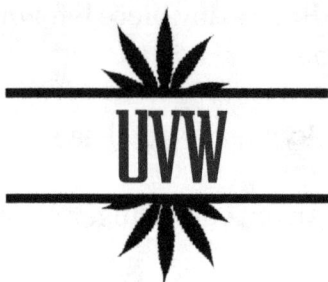

Weed: Slang for ganja.

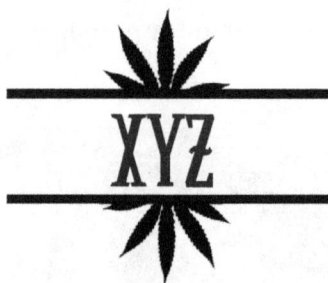

XYZ

Zip: An ounce of ganja. The word comes from a brand of sandwich bag that is often used to package an ounce of ganja.

USES OF GANJA

Medicinal

Ganja has been medically prescribed and recommended for relief from the symptoms of many diseases and conditions. Some of these are:

- Glaucoma
- Anxiety
- General nausea and vomiting
- Pain caused by structural or psycho-physiological disorders
- Neuropathy (diseases affecting the nerves)
- Migraine headaches
- Muscular spasticity and limb pain (like multiple sclerosis)
- Treatment for symptoms of AIDS
- Treatment for symptoms of movement disorders like Tourette's syndrome and Parkinson's disease

- A chemical in ganja helps to stop cancer from spreading
- May slow the progression of Alzheimer's disease
- Appears to lesson the side effects from treating hepatitis C and increase treatment effectiveness
- Can help with inflammatory bowel diseases
- Helps to relieve arthritis discomfort
- Helps people suffering from PTSD

Recreational

There is much evidence of the recreational use of ganja throughout history, and it is massively popular across the globe. When used responsibly by adults, there are no adverse economic, legal, social or health consequences. The use of ganja is a staple in all classes and layers of society. More than one former president of the United States has admitted using ganja. Some of the benefits of using ganja recreationally include:

- Helps one to relax
- Can open up one's mind to new ideas and possibilities
- Smoking ganja helps people to experience things like music and films more intensely
- Can spur creativity in those who are artistically inclined
- Can help one to get in touch with one's higher self spiritually *(no pun intended)*

Products

Hemp, also known as industrial hemp, is a variety of the sativa plant that is grown specifically for the industrial uses of its derived products. It was used in China and the Middle East from as far back as 8000 BC. It can be refined into a number of commercial items such as:

- Textiles
- Clothing
- Paper
- Canvas
- Boat sails
- Animal feed
- Paint
- Biodegradable plastics
- Oil based products
- Bio fuel

Strains

Ganja plants come in both the male and female variety, and vary in size and stature. There are two widely acknowledged strains: sativa and indica.

Sativa

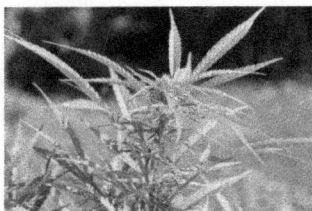

Many people prefer to smoke this strain as it has an invigorating and stimulating effect on the user. This is the ideal strain for someone who wants to have a smoke in the morning and he/she is going to be active and energetic during the course of the day. Sativa plants grow quite large, capable of reaching up to fifteen feet, and the leaves are dainty, long and narrow.

Indica

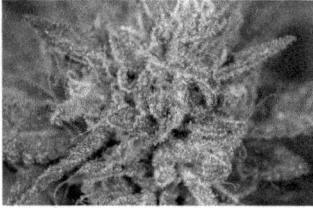

This strain tends to have a sedating effect on the user and puts the entire body into a deep relaxing state. The effects of this strain tend to be more sedating than stimulating. Indica plants usually grow between three to six feet tall, and being that it is a short plant, it is perfect for indoor growing. The buds and flowers on the indica plant tend to grow very close to each other.

Famous Proponents

There has been a lot of propaganda dispensed throughout the years about ganja and the use of it, and one of the most widespread is that those who are heavy ganja smokers are lazy and unproductive. Nothing could be further from the truth. Here are some ganja proponents, from actors to singers to businessmen who have all been extremely successful in their careers while indulging heavily in nature's most dynamic herb.

Bob Marley

The great, late reggae legend advocated for ganja throughout his adult life, citing the herb's greatness.

Seth Rogen

The comedic actor has publicly said he smokes ganja every day and tends to portray stoners in his movies as funny and cool characters.

Snoop Dog

Through his music and lifestyle, the legendary rapper has long let the world know about his love for ganja. He has also invested in it, having released his own line of ganja called Leafs by Snoop.

Willie Nelson

The country music veteran is a heavy ganja smoker and has his own line of ganja products called Willie's Reserve.

Rihanna

The pop star has been quite open about her ganja use, often taking pictures or making short videos of her smoking the herb.

Oliver Stone

The director has smoked great ganja all over the world and has been a regular ganja smoker since his days as an infantryman in Vietnam in the late 1960s.

Morgan Freeman

The veteran actor is a public voice advocating for the legalization of ganja, and has cited using it for fibromyalgia pain, saying that it is the only thing that gives him relief.

Martha Stewart

The American businesswoman and television personality is a self-proclaimed expert at rolling joints.

Hugh Hefner

The late businessman was a ganja smoker and said that smoking helped to put him in touch with the realm of the senses.

Phil Jackson

The legendary basketball coach spoke frankly about his ganja use in his memoir about his playing days in the NBA.

Lady Gaga

The pop star smokes a lot of ganja when writing music.

Jokes & Mantras

One of the pleasant effects of smoking ganja is the unbridled joy you feel when you find something funny. The uncontrollable laughter, the shaking, the tears running from your eyes, it's an epic experience laughing while stoned. Here are a few popular ganja related jokes and mantras.

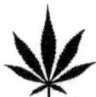

A ganja smoker calls the fire department. "Please hurry!" he says. "My house is on fire!"
The dispatcher asks, "How do we get there?"
The man replies, "In a big red truck, duh!"

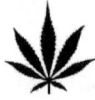

A narcotics detective stopped at a farm and said to the farmer, "I need to inspect your farm for illegally growing ganja."

The farmer replied, "Ok, but don't go in that field over there..."

The detective didn't take kindly to that. "Sir, I have the authority of the government with me!" he shouted and removed his badge. "See this damn badge?" he continued, waving the badge in the farmer's face. "This badge means I am allowed to go wherever I wish on any land as long as I suspect criminal activity! No questions asked! Have I made myself clear? Do you understand me?"

The farmer apologized and went about his chores. A short time later, he heard loud screams and looked up to see the narcotics detective running for his life, being chased by the farmer's huge mean bull. With every step the bull was gaining on the detective, and it seemed inevitable that he was going to get gored before he reached safety. The detective was beyond terrified.

The farmer quickly threw down his tools, ran to the fence and yelled at the top of his lungs, "Your badge! Show him your damn badge!"

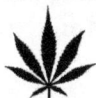

A ganja smoker and a genius are sitting on a bench waiting for a bus. Bored, the genius says to the ganja smoker, "Hey, tell you what, I'll ask you a question and if you don't know the answer, you have to give me five dollars. But if you ask me a question and I don't know the answer, I have to give you fifty dollars."

The ganja smoker replies, "Alright, man."

The genius asks, "What is the Pythagorean Theory?"

The ganja smoker responds, "I don't know."

He gives the genius five dollars and then asks, "What has three legs going up a hill and four legs going down?"

The genius thinks really hard and then finally gives up. He admits he doesn't know and gives the ganja smoker fifty dollars.

"So what is the answer?" he asks.

"I don't know," the ganja smoker replies, and hands the genius five dollars.

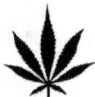

Police officer: "How high are you?"

Stoner: "No, officer. It's 'Hi, how are you?'"

Q: What does a mermaid smoke?
A: Seaweed

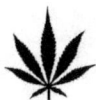

Q: How do you know when you have smoked enough ganja?

A: When you start looking for the directions on how to use the lighter.

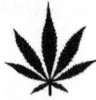

*   Alcohol kills. Weed chills.

*   Haters bring drama. Stoners bring ganja.

*   Don't drink and drive. Park and spark.

*   Under the influence but above the ignorance.

Top Ten Ganja Songs & Movies

Pop culture has always had a love affair with ganja. From music to movies, millions of people worldwide have bonded using the magical rope of the world's most popular herb.

Songs

- Alkaline - Direction (2016)

- Vybz Kartel - Sen' On (2003)

- Rick James - Mary Jane (1978)

- Rihanna - James Joint (2016)

- D.R.A.M. - Broccoli (2016)

- Young Thug - Stoner (2014)

- ❀ Afroman - Because I Got High (2000)

- ❀ Mighty Diamonds - Pass The Kouchie (1982)

- ❀ D' Angelo - Brown Sugar (1995)

- ❀ Peter Tosh - Legalize It (1976)

Movies

- Half Baked (1998)

- Friday (1995)

- Fast Times at Ridgemont High (1982)

- Pineapple Express (2008)

- How High (2001)

- Up In Smoke (1978)

- Cheech and Chong's Next Movie (1980)

- Dazed and Confused (1993)

- Saving Grace (2000)

- Ted (2012)

Quotes

"I think people need to be educated to the fact that marijuana is not a drug. Marijuana is an herb and a flower. God put it here. If He put it here and He wants it to grow, what gives the government the right to say that God is wrong?"
~ Willie Nelson

"Herb is the healing of a nation, alcohol is the destruction."   **~ Bob Marley**

"Is marijuana addictive? Yes, in the sense that most of the really pleasant things in life are worth endlessly repeating."
~ Richard Neville

"Instead of taking five or six of the prescriptions, I decided to go a natural route and smoke marijuana."
~ Melissa Etheridge